# Natural Remedies For Beginners

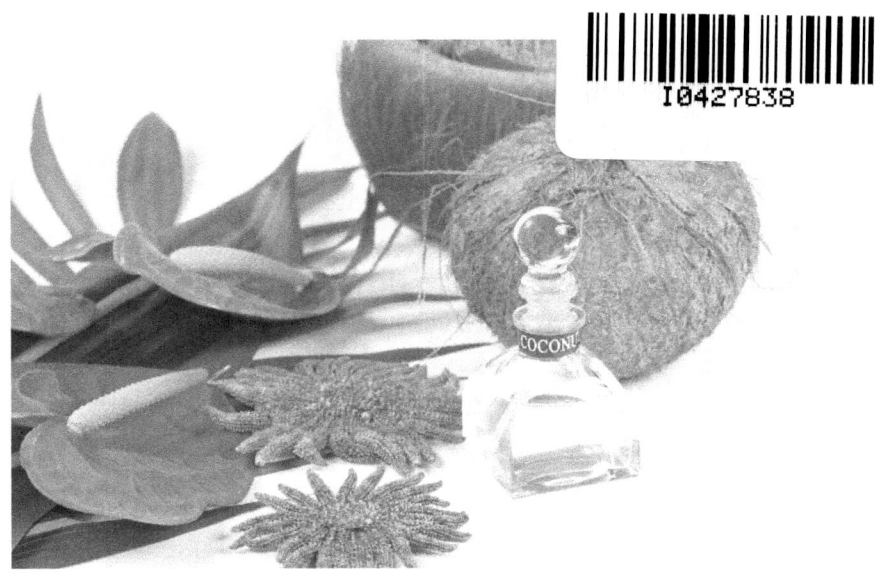

# How To Heal Protect and Beautify Yourself Without Prescriptions

## By Dr Brad Turner

## Disclaimer

This book is intended to be a general guide, to raise awareness, and to help people make informed decisions in the context of their own personal circumstance. As everybody's circumstances are different, so are the remedies you should seek. While many of the recommendations in this book can be applied by almost anybody regardless of their conditions they are not intended to and should not be relied upon to replace personal medical advice.

The author accepts no responsibility for any loss or injury, be it personal or financial, as a result for the use or misuse of the information in this book. If you have any doubts or concerns after reading this book, please speak to a doctor or other qualified person before taking any actions.

## From The Author

Thank you for taking the time to read this book. As an author, I understand the importance of creating books which my readers will find both enjoyable and informative. If you have the time and feel generous, please don't hesitate to leave an honest review of this book.........Dr Brad Turner.

# Contents

## Introduction

## Chapter 1
### Remedies For Daily Ailments
Heartburn
Joint Pain
Headache
Menstrual Cramps
Yeast Infection
Muscle Pain

## Chapter 2
### Remedies To Treat Skin & External Ailments
Sunburn
Toenail Fungus
Puffy Eyes
Rash
Eczema
Psoriasis

## Chapter 3
### Gastrointestinal Remedies
Diarrhoea
Constipation
Bloating & Gas
Nausea

# Introduction

Today, many advances have been made in the field of medical science, which resulted to the formulation, distribution, and widespread use of modern medicinal drugs. The people's faith in these drugs have become so strong that any alternative cure for any kind of disease or ailment have been looked down upon, and the use of natural remedies have been subjected to this prejudice.

It is not until a few decades ago that awareness of the negative effects of chemical drugs and substances as cure to common and serious illnesses have started to break into the zeitgeist of the times. By that time, many people have also started to realize the importance of 'going back to the basics' and looking to Mother Nature for cure instead.

Little do people know that the products that they rely on are in one way or another made up of plants and things from nature, and that humans, even animals, have been using medicinal plants, techniques, and other natural remedies for thousands of years. The fact that people from the older times have life spans longer than that of today's people serves as evidence of the effectiveness of natural remedies.

Compared to modern day drugs, which have been derived from artificial and chemical sources, natural remedies have more benefits to offer. For one, natural remedies are cheaper. Making your own natural and organic concoction, powder, or paste, for common diseases and ailments is far more cost-efficient than buying those over the counter medicines that are very pricey, even crazily expensive at times. Other than being cheaper, another reason why natural remedies are better than over the counter medicines is that they can be made in the comfort of your own home, most of the time using ingredients that can be easily found in your kitchen and garden or are readily available in your local market. Another thing is that natural remedies do not have chemical or synthetic ingredients in them, and thus have lesser risks of side effects. Lastly, because our ancestors have been using these natural remedies for a very long time, our bodies are already accustomed to the substances in them, reducing chances of allergies or adverse reactions.

However, you must still be careful in handling the things that are part of your regimen, especially plants or plant parts. Although they can be equally effective as commercial synthetic drugs, they are still plants after all which have natural toxins to protect them. But no worries, by knowing the right amount to use, what part to use, and how to properly prepare whatever natural concoctions you want to make, you can easily make yourself natural remedies, which not only are cost-efficient, practical and effective, but also safe.

The following chapters will guide you through a collection of common ailments and afflictions and their corresponding effective natural remedies that you can easily make on your own.

# Chapter 1
## Daily Ailment Remedies

## Heartburn

The problem with heartburn is basically the stomach acid scalding your oesophagus. That is why most of the effective natural remedies for heartburn involve neutralizing this acid. Here is a list of the most common way for naturally and effectively alleviating heartburn:

- **Drink tea.** Teas, specifically those made from chamomile or ginger, can help buffer the acids. For the chamomile tea, just boil a cup of water, mix it with either a chamomile tea bag or a teaspoon of dried petals of chamomile and let it steep for 2 to 3 minutes. Drink an hour before you sleep. For the ginger tea, just have 3 to 4 slices of ginger simmered in 1 to 2 cups of water. Drink 20 to 30 minutes before each meal.

- **Eat apple, banana and mustard**. These are known acid neutralizers. Have some before, during, or after meals.

- **Drink fat free milk or skim milk**. The calcium, which is abundantly present in milk is one known and proven acid 'buffer' and is, in fact, the active ingredient of a number of antacids. Make sure its fat free, as fat can encourage more acid production.

- **Chew gum.** Although gum is not essentially a natural product, chewing gum has been proven and tested to address heartburn. It is not the gum itself, but the saliva produced when chewing that is effective in neutralizing stomach acid. It also helps the acids recede back to the stomach and out of your system. Try chewing a piece of gum after meals, particularly those that are sugar-free.

## Joint Pain

For joint pains, the most common and effective remedies focus on pain relief and addressing inflammation. To ease and prevent joint paints, you can have:

- **Turmeric tea.** Turmeric is a known anti-inflammatory agent. In a cup of boiling water, just add half a teaspoon of turmeric powder or 3 slices of turmeric. Let it simmer for 10 minutes, strain, transfer in a cup, and drink with a few tablespoons of honey.

- **Eucalyptus and peppermint ointment**. Just combine 8 drops of eucalyptus oil and 8 drops of peppermint oil with 2 drops of olive oil or grape seed oil in a small tinted container. Apply on affected joints.

- **Dandelion leaves**. You can put in 2 to 3 teaspoons of dandelion leaves (fresh) in a cup of hot boiling water. Let cool and drink, preferably with two servings a day. You can also put in fresh dandelion leaves in your salads.

- **White willow tea.** The bark of the White willow is like nature's 'aspirin'. Just add in 2 teaspoons of the powdered bark in a cup of boiling water. Let it simmer for 10 minutes and then let it sleep for another 20

minutes away from heat. Drink two times a day
.

- **Extra virgin coconut oil.** EVOO is both anti-inflammatory and a pain-reliever. There are two ways to use EVOO. You can just use it as an ointment, or you can take in 3 tablespoons per day.

## Headache

For headaches, the best natural remedies are:

- **Peppermint and Eucalyptus ointment.** Just like in joint pains, these oils can help soothe the pain. Just follow the instructions on how to make this ointment in the Joint Pain section.

- **Ginger tea.** Ginger can also alleviate headache pains and help ease nausea. Instructions on how to make ginger tea can be found in the Heartburn section.

- **Feverfew tea.** Feverfew is a common plant that is known to help reduce the pressure in blood vessels and also has anti-inflammatory and pain relieving properties.  Just add 1 tablespoon of feverfew flowers, fresh or dried, in a cup of boiling water. Let it steep for ten minutes. Drink once a day, preferably half a cup in the morning and half a cup in the afternoon or evening.

- **Water.** Water is perhaps the simplest and most effective headache reliever out there, since most headaches occur because you are not hydrated enough.

# Menstrual Cramps

Menstrual cramps are a monthly burden for all women. To help alleviate this ailment, you can take in some of the following:

- **Chamomile tea.** Chamomile is also a known pain reliever. The recipe for a relaxing cup of chamomile tea can be found in the Heartburn section.

- **Ginger tea.** To ease the pain of cramps, you can take in a cup of ginger tea. The recipe can be found in the Heartburn section.

- **Fennel tea.** Fennel is helpful in improving the blood flow in the uterus, thus reducing cramping. Just mix in a teaspoon of ground fennel seeds in a cup of boiling water, let it steep for 5 to 6 minutes, strain and drink while still warm.

- **Water.** Cramps become more painful when the body is dehydrated. Just drink 6 to 8 glasses of water a day and you will find the pain from your menstrual cramps easing off.

# Yeast Infection

Yeast infections are usually caused by a species of yeast called Candida albicans, which is a fungus. To cure yeast infection, you can have the following:

- **Tea tree oil ointment**. Tea tree oil has is widely used treatment for yeast infections because of its antifungal and antiseptic properties. Just dilute three drops of the essential oil in one third cup water. Soak a cotton swab or tampon and apply in affected area.

- **Yoghurt**. Yoghurt (live culture) has good bacteria that can help fight off fungal infections. Just apply natural and unsweetened yoghurt in affected area. It will also provide a cooling and relieving sensation.

- **Cranberry juice**. This juice has always been recommended for bacterial and fungal infections. Drink a glass of cranberry juice a day to balance the pH level of your urine and cure the infection.

- **Garlic**. Garlic is a natural effective antibacterial. You can add fresh garlic in your every meal. Not only can it fight off infection, it can also help your immune system.

## Muscle Pain

Whenever you do any strenuous activity, muscle pains surely come after. To relieve muscle pains, you can use the following:

- **Hot pepper poultice/rubs.** Hot pepper has capsaicin, which is a natural pain reliever. Just mix in half a teaspoon of cayenne pepper powder to EVOO or warm virgin coconut oil. Apply in affected area and keep it away from sensitive areas like the eyes and mouth.

- **Use essential oils.** Using essential oils like eucalyptus and peppermint as ointments (recipe in Joint Pain section) can help relax the muscles and alleviate pain. You can also use one or a combination of two of some essential oils like lemongrass, basil, lavender, marjoram and chamomile, in EVOO or coconut oil.

- **Apple cider vinegar.** ACV is a muscle pain reliever. You can soak a cloth with AVC and apply it in the affected area for 20 to 25 minutes, and apply again every three hours.

# Chapter 2
## Remedies To Treat Skin & External Ailments

## Sunburn

Sunburn can be pretty nasty. Not only can it wreak havoc to your looks and leave ugly patterns on your skin, it can also give you a heck of a sting. If you have sunburns, the following can be useful to you:

- **Honey**. Honey is a wonder from nature. Among its numerous health benefits, it can also help heal sunburned skin faster and provide a soothing effect. Just apply honey on the affected area, but make sure that it is organic as it is more effective that way.

- **Aloe vera.** Aloe has always been a popular natural remedy for burned skin. It can get rid of the pain and give a nice cool and soothing feeling. Just get a plump aloe leaf, slit it in the centre and spread it out, then gently rub the gel on the burned skin.

- **Milk**. The proteins in the milk help cover the burn and help the skin cells heal faster. It can also provide a soothing feeling when chilled. Just soak clean cotton gauze or cloth with chilled milk, apply in the affected area, and leave it there until it is no longer cool. Reapply again if necessary.

- **Mint and black tea solution.** While mint naturally gives off a cooling sensation, tea has theobromine and tannic acid, which helps reduce pain and help skin heal faster. Just let one black tea bag and 1 cup of crushed mint leaves steep in hot water for 1 hour. Strain the liquid, chill it, and apply on the skin with a clean cotton gauze or cloth.

# Toenail Fungus

Not only are the manifestations of toenail fungus not easy on the eyes, it can also lead to more serious problems, like your nails falling off. The following natural remedies can help you get rid of this.

- **Tea tree oil and orange oil ointments**. Like yeast infections, tea tree oil and orange oil is very effective in solving other fungal problems because of its anti-fungal and anti-bacterial properties. Just mix in half a teaspoon of orange oil, a teaspoon of tea tree oil, and a teaspoon of EVOO. Soak a clean cotton ball with the mixture and apply on the affected area.

- **Coconut oil.** The fatty acids in coconut oil help disintegrate the fungi. To do so, just soak in cotton ball with the oil and apply where necessary. Use three times a day.

- **Apple cider vinegar or white vinegar.** Because vinegars are alkaline, it upsets the acidic environment that the fungi thrive in. To treat toenail fungus with this, you only have to soak your feet in a litre of water and a cup of vinegar for 10 to 15 minutes.

# Puffy Eyes

Puffy eyes from crying are an inconvenience, especially when you have to go out afterwards. To easily reduce the puffiness of your eyes, you can opt to use the following:

- **Cucumbers**. Cucumbers are very popular as solutions to eye bags and puffy eyes. They have anti-inflammatory properties that help reduce swelling. Slice a fresh large cucumber into quarter inch thick slices and place them over both of your eyes for 10 minutes.

- **Potato bags**. The starch in potatoes also has anti-inflammatory properties. To make use of potatoes, just clean a whole potato and shred them to small pieces. Get two small clothes and use them to wrap a handful of shredded potatoes. Place each of them on your eyes for 5 to 6 minutes

- **Egg whites**. Egg whites have properties that help tighten the skin. To use egg whites, you only have to combine the whites of 2 eggs and beat them until they make stiff peaks. Spread the whites under your eyes until they are dry, and then remove it.

- **Tea bags**. Teas have caffeine that helps constrict blood vessels and tones down the puffiness. Steep two tea bags in a cup of water, remove the bags and chill them in the fridge. Place the bags under your eyes for 1 minute.

# Rash

Skin rashes are a nuisance and a source of great pain. To help cure rashes you can do the following:

- **Use aloe vera**. Aloe is not only effective in treating burns, but rashes as well. The soothing effect of aloe can help keep away the itch and it also helps make the skin healthy. Use and apply aloe leaves the same way as you use it in treating Sunburns.

- **Have an oatmeal bath**. Oatmeal has chemicals that protect the skin and have anti-inflammatory properties that help soothe irritation. To make an oatmeal bath, you only have to mix in a cup of uncooked oats in your tub filled with water. Soak in the tub for 20 to 30 minutes.

- **Olive oil**. Olive oil, particularly EVOO, has anti-inflammatory properties as well as moisturizing effect. Both of these properties help soothe and heal skin rashes. Just soak in a cotton ball with olive oil and apply on the rashes.

# Eczema

Not only is eczema very agonizing, it also stops you from wearing your favourite clothes and can be source of embarrassment. To treat eczema, these natural remedies can be used:

- **Yoghurt**. The good bacteria in yoghurts, especially those with live culture, help treat eczema. You can eat 2 to 3 cups of unfrozen yoghurt daily, and at the same time apply them on the skin.

- **Pickles and other fermented foods**. Pickled foods are alkaline, thus it can adjust the pH level of the body to fight off eczema. You can add dill pickles, sauerkraut or kimchi in your everyday diet, and at the same time, use and apply the extracts or juice externally on the affected area of your skin.

- **Avocado, olive oil and aloe vera poultice**. All three have beneficial properties, which have always been used to treat skin diseases. To make the poultice, combine the pulp of a whole avocado, the gel inside an aloe leaf, and a quarter of a cup of EVOO. Mix in a food processor and put in the fridge until firm. Apply in affected area.

## Psoriasis

Of all the common skin diseases, psoriasis is one of the most painful and uncomfortable. Some of the most effective natural remedies to treat psoriasis include:

- **Oatmeal.** Like rashes, psoriasis can also be treated using the power of oatmeal. You can use oats in two ways, one is by having an oatmeal bath (the recipe can be found in the Rashes section) and another is by using an oatmeal paste. To make the cream, just combine a cup of oats and enough water to form some kind of paste. Apply in the affected skin.

- **Tea tree oil**. Just like most skin ailments, tea tree oil can also be used for psoriasis. Use it the same way as you treat Toenail fungus.

- **Olive oil**. Olive oil also is very effective for this skin ailment, as it soothes inflammation, reduces pain or itchiness, and moisturizes the skin. Soak cotton ball in olive oil and apply gently on the skin.

# Chapter 3
## Gastrointestinal Remedies

## Diarrhoea

Diarrhoea, if not addressed quickly can become a serious inconvenience to you, and worse, can make you dehydrated and weak. To stop diarrhoea and prevent it from worsening, you can use the following:

- **Fenugreek seeds.** Fenugreek is consisted of a lot of fibre, which can help thicken the stool. Just add half a teaspoon of fenugreek seeds in a glass of cold water. Drink three times a day.

- **Chamomile tea.** Chamomile has a natural property that eases inflammation in the intestinal tract and also helps the colon relax. Recipe of the chamomile tea can be found in the Heartburn section.

- **Orange peel tea.** The rind of oranges has been a common and known treatment for diarrhoea as it helps improve one's digestion and thus quickly wash away the bad bacteria that cause diarrhoea out of the body. Just peel off an entire orange and mix the peel with 2 cups of boiling water. Then, steep it for a few minutes or until the mixture is lukewarm.

- **Salt and sugar drink**. Dissolve half a teaspoon of salt and a teaspoon of sugar in glass of water, and drink several times a day. Other than water, which will keep you from being dehydrated, this solution also helps restore electrolytes lost from your body.

- **Yoghurt.** Yoghurt helps bring good bacteria back into your colon, which can help in stopping diarrhoea. Eat 3 cups of yoghurt per day, preferably natural and unflavoured ones.

# Constipation

Like diarrhoea, constipation is a great hassle and a source of great pain. It can sometimes even lead to more serious complications. The following natural remedies can help you deal with constipation.

- **Olive oil**. Taking in oils are effective in constipation as they are natural lubricants. They help smooth out the digestion process. Olive oil is not the tastiest constipation remedy out there, so you can take it with some juice. Just mix in a tablespoon of EVOO with half a teaspoon of lemon juice or a whole glass of lemon juice.

- **Flax seed oil**. Just like EVOO, flax seed oil is effective for constipation. You can take it in the same way you take in olive oil, either with a glass of lemon juice or orange juice.

- **Prunes**. Prunes and also prune juice are a popular and effective way to cure constipation. Not only do they have so much fibre, they are also rich in sorbitol, a substance, which can help make your stool soft. Drink two glasses a day, one in the morning and one in the evening.

- **Lemon**. Lemon is rich in citric acid and acts like a stimulant for your digestive system. It also helps rid your body of toxins and wash your colons. Just squeeze in fresh lemon in a cup of warm water. You can feel its effects within a few minutes.

- **Dandelion tea**. Dandelion leaves are a very effective remedy for constipation as it is a natural laxative and is also an antioxidant. To make dandelion tea, just refer to the section on Joint Pain.

## Bloating & Gas

Bloating and flatulence is not a very serious ailment, except when you release gas in the most unfortunate of times. But these embarrassing things should not be taken lightly, especially that they can be signs of much more serious conditions.

- **Caraway seeds**. Caraway seeds have long been used to help pass out gas. If you feel bloated and can't seem to expel the gas inside, you can much on caraway seeds (just a pinch) or crackers with caraway seeds every morning.

- **Anise seeds**. Anise, just like caraway seeds, is an effective carminative which help let gas out of your body. It also has substances, which are anti-spasmodic. You can also chew on a pinch of anise seeds regularly until you pass gas.

- **Ginger.** Yes, its ginger again. Ginger is also another good carminative, due to two substances present in it, specifically shogaols and gingerol. They also help relieve inflammation and relax the colon. You can either munch on small pieces throughout the day or have a teaspoon of grated ginger before your meals. You can also enjoy it as tea (recipe of ginger tea can be found in section on Headaches).

- **Peppermint tea**. And yes, peppermint enters into the spotlight again, and you're going to see more of it, just like ginger. Anyway, the menthol in peppermint has antispasmodic properties, and can also serve as a soothing agent for the nerves and make the pain less miserable. To prepare the tea, you only have to steep a tablespoon of dried peppermint leaves in a cup of boiling water for 15 minutes. Strain and drink when warm.

- **Pumpkin**. Pumpkin is one effective way of reducing the production of gas during digestion. To do this, you should take in a cup of pumpkin along with your meals. You can have them in whatever form you want, mashed, steamed, or as a dessert.

## Nausea

Having nausea gives you both discomfort and hassle, especially when you won't be able to do the things you want and need to do. That is why though nausea, especially those caused by gastrointestinal complications, is not that serious and will just go away by itself; it still has to be treated right away. You can do this by:

- **Inhaling lemon extract**. The citrusy smell of lemons has been found to help ease nausea. With just a slice of lemon, you can relieve yourself of that nauseating feeling by inhaling its scent. Do this until the discomfort has been quelled.

- **Eat bread**. Yes, the simple eating of bread is effective in easing nausea, especially one that is caused by acid in the stomach, as the bread helps to absorb it and decrease the concentration of acid.

- **Take in ginger**. Ginger has many medicinal benefits, as what you may have known by now, and that includes alleviating nausea caused by acid. You can either take a cup or two of ginger tea, or a broth with a ginger base. You can also chew on a small piece until the feeling goes away.

- **Peppermint**. The scent and cooling effect of peppermint has been known to have a great effect on alleviating nausea. You can enjoy it as tea or use it as an ointment. Just apply a bit of peppermint oil on your gums, and it will do the trick. At the same time, you can also inhale the scent for it to have a stronger effect.

# Chapter 4
## Mental & Neurological Remedies

## Anxiety

Anxiety isn't as simple as being fidgety and nervous. It can affect you in ways that can also be detrimental to your physical health, especially due to high cortisol levels in your system and insomnia. To help address insomnia, you can have the following natural remedies:

- **Chamomile tea.** Chamomile has been mentioned in this book quite a few times, which is not surprising since chamomile has a wide range of health benefits, including the alleviation of anxiety. If you feel a bout of anxiety, have yourself a cup of chamomile tea, and for insomnia, drink decaffeinated chamomile tea 30 minutes before going to sleep.

- **Omega 3 fatty acids.** These fatty acids, mostly found in fishes like tuna and salmon, have been found to help prevent the occurrence of anxiety or help alleviate it. Other than getting it from your diet, there are oil capsules available in the market. You have to take in not less than 2.5 mg of it per day.

- **Passionflower.** This natural remedy has already been used in various countries for a long time as an answer to anxiety, as it is a natural sedative. For a more relaxed feeling and a restful sleep, have a tablespoon of it and steep in a cup of boiling water for around 10 minutes. Drink 30 minutes before bedtime. But remember to not take this if you are pregnant.

- **Lavender.** Lavender is not just easy on the eyes, but to the mind as well. It has natural properties that help calm down nerves and relieve stress. For a more relaxed feeling, get yourself a whiff of lavender oil or spray diluted lavender oil in your room.

## Mild Depression

When the word 'depression' comes to mind, most people immediately think about doctors and medications. But you don't have to look to medicinal drugs for answers right away, when you already have the solution inside your own home. These effective natural remedies can be found in the list below. The deal with addressing depression is to increase serotonin levels in your system, a hormone that is even dubbed as the 'happy hormone'.

- **Pumpkin seed**. There are three important substances in pumpkin seeds that help depression: fats (the healthy type), magnesium, and L-trytophan. Together they keep the chemical balance in the brain in check and increase serotonin levels up to its normal point. For the dosage, remember that a heaping cup of pumpkin seeds a day can keep depression away.

- **Chamomile tea**. Like ginger and peppermint, chamomile is a regular in this book, which is not a surprise because of its wide range of benefits. Like in anxiety, chamomile tea mostly aids when it comes to sleeping problems. Take a nice warm cup half an hour before you go to bed to help you relax and have a peaceful sleep.

- **Green tea**. Though caffeine is a no-no for depression, the caffeine in green tea is balanced out by a compound called L-theanine, which is helpful in clearing the havoc of transmitters in your brain and also induce production of dopamine, which is another helpful hormone in alleviating depression. Unlike chamomile tea, have your green tea during breakfast so that in can help you for the day.

- **Banana**. This fruit has become popular as an effective way of increasing serotonin levels. However, while bananas do have serotonin, they don't actually have a direct effect on the brain. It is the high amount of Vitamin B6 in them that aid your brain to make more of its own serotonin. Eat once a day, preferably before meals. You can also have it with spinach and mackerel in your meals as they also have high concentrations of B Vitamins.

# Insomnia

Insomnia becomes a problem when it starts to affect the physiological health of a person and when it hinders normal day-to-day functioning. It is also not an exclusive condition, as it can also manifest together with or as a symptom of other ailments like anxiety and depression. That is why you can also find that some remedies used for these conditions can also be applied in treating insomnia.

- **Melatonin**. Melatonin is the hormone that helps regulate your sleeping pattern or your 'circadian rhythm'. Though there are already available melatonin supplements in the market, there are also many natural sources of this hormone that can be derives from plants. These include feverfew and fenugreek seeds. You can enjoy feverfew as tea (recipe in the Headache section) 30 minutes before you sleep.

- **Tart cherries**. Another plant product that can help increase melatonin content in the brain is tart cherry. You can either take it in as juice, about a glass of it, twice a day, one in the morning and another 30 minutes before you go to sleep.

- **Valerian**. Valerian, specifically its roots, has long been used as a sedative and as an aid for sleeping, which is why it can also be used not only for insomnia but also for anxiety. You can take valerian root in capsule form, or as tea. Just let a teaspoon of the root (dried) steep in a mug of boiling water for more or less 15 minutes. Strain, and enjoy 30 minutes before sleeping.

- **Lavender aromatherapy**. The scent of lavender has always been lauded for its calming and relaxing effect, which is why it is also used for anxiety. To use lavender for insomnia, just spray your room, your bed and pillows, with diluted lavender oil.

- **Chamomile tea**. The relaxing effect of chamomile tea is effective for inducing drowsiness and sleep. Have a cup of warm chamomile tea 30 minutes before you want to go to sleep.

# Vertigo

Having vertigo is not only a simple inconvenience and source of great discomfort; it can also be downright dangerous and can result to malfunctioning.

- **Ginger.** Ginger is good for many ailments, and vertigo is one of them. It has natural properties that are proven to ease the nauseating feeling associated with movement, which is the case in vertigo most of the time. And it also helps improve blood pressure and circulation. When dizziness comes, have a cup of tea, or chew on a few small pieces of ginger root. It would also be good if you have tea and ginger root in your diet every day.

- **Gingko biloba**. Many people with vertigo have benefited from gingko biloba, as it has properties that help improve blood circulation to the brain, bringing with it loads of oxygen. There are numbers of gingko biloba products sold in the market today that come in pills or capsules. You only have to take 120 mg of it per day for not more than three months.

- **Feverfew**. Feverfew has properties that help regulate blood pressure, which is helpful in alleviating dizziness and vertigo. You can enjoy feverfew as tea (recipe in the Headache section) everyday, half a cup each morning and evening.

# Chapter 5
## Natural Remedies For Mild Infections

## Common Cold

The cold is perhaps one of the simplest and less dangerous ailments that one can contract every now and then, but it is also one of the most debilitating. Unfortunately, a cure for cold has not been discovered, and what we can only do is alleviate the symptoms, which actually make the cold inconvenient, like congestion, and help the immune system fight back.

- **Mullein**. Mullein tea has natural properties that help ease nasal congestion by inducing your body to expel the accumulated mucus. To enjoy it as a tea, you only have to steep a teaspoon of dried mullein leaves and a teaspoon of its dried flowers in a cup of boiling water for 15 minutes. Strain properly as it has tiny hairs that can irritate your mouth and throat. Use not more than thrice a day.

- **Chicken noodle soup**. The chicken noodle soup myth is true; it can help you get over your cold fast. The secret of this soup is in its ingredients, which have been proven to strengthen the immune system, clear out congestion, and soothe irritation, such as onions, celery, carrots, and hot broth. You can make your soup in any way you want, just don't use the ones sold in stores.

- **Garlic**. Garlic has antibacterial and anti-inflammatory properties that help clear your airways from congestion. Include a lot of garlic in your meals, or have a garlic tea by boiling 5 garlic cloves in a cup of water and letting it steep for 5 to 6 minutes.

## Coughs

Cough usually presents itself together or after a bout of cold, making it more unbearable. It's embarrassing too, when you have to cough and cough uncontrollably in public places. To do away with cough, do the following:

- **Have honey**. Research has shown that honey is a very effective demulcent, forming a soothing protection on the throat lining that lessens irritation. Just take 3 tablespoons of pure organic honey a day.

- **Take ginger tea**. Ginger is a natural expectorant, effective in expelling phlegm out of the body. Have it when it's still steaming hot.

- **Drink thyme tea**. Thyme has components that help relax and soothe the lungs and air passageways. Have four sprigs of fresh thyme and pound them slightly. Let them steep in a glass of boiling water for 15 minutes and enjoy three times a day.

- **Inhale steam with essential oils**. Steam helps break down mucous and stubborn phlegm, while essential oils like those from peppermint and eucalyptus help clear airways and eliminate the virus. Just have a bowl of steaming water with two drops of peppermint oil and 2 drops of eucalyptus oil. Place your face over the bowl and inhale the steam, but make sure it's not hot enough to scald your face. This is effective for colds, too.

## Sore Throat

Having sore throat is painful, and it also becomes a hindrance when most of your day requires you to talk. Colds, cough, and sore throat basically belong to the same family of ailments, which is why remedies for the other two is also effective for sore throat. Other natural remedies that help alleviate sore throat include:

- **Apple cider vinegar**. AVC has an acidity that is able to kill the bacteria residing in your throat. Just mix in a teaspoon of it in a cup of warm water and drink, or you can gargle before swallowing it.

- **Warm salt gargle**. Gargling water with salt helps bring down the swelling of the membranes of your throat and reduce the pain, as salt brings out water from them. Mix in half a teaspoon of salt in a cup of warm water and gargle it thrice a day.

- **Pomegranate juice**. Pomegranate has an astringent property that helps reduce swelling, and thus decrease pain. You can have two glasses of organic unsweetened pomegranate juice a day, and make sure to gargle it before swallowing.

# First Aid Ointment

In accidents, you always immediately look for creams and ointments that are synthetic and made up of chemicals. But even without them, you can still perform first aid treatment with just your pantry and nature as your medicinal kit.

# Plantain Ointment

Plantain may just be a weed to others but it has amazing properties that are perfect for first aid treatment of bites, stings, wounds, allergies, rashes, sunburns and other skin problems. To make plantain ointment, all you need to have is the following:

- 4 oz. olive oil infused with dried plantain leaf
- 1 oz. Beeswax
- 5 drops Vitamin E (oil)
- 3 drops of peppermint oil
- 2 Mason jars

# How To Prepare

1.    For the infused olive oil, fill a dry Mason jar (a quart) with dried plantain leaves and the olive oil. Tightly seal. Place the jar in a crock-pot with a layer of towel at the bottom; fill it with water reaching half the jar. Set it to warm for two days

2.    For making the ointment, pour beeswax and strained oil in a pan over low heat. Stir, and remove when melted. Add the Vitamin E oil and the peppermint oil, and stir. Transfer to a dry Mason jar and let stand for a day to harden. Use when needed.

# Conclusion

Congratulations! You now have read the last page in this book and by now you probably are already armed with the helpful and relevant information on natural remedies that you can easily use and make.

But before you go about using these natural remedies, there are still some considerations that you have to make. To be on the safe side of things, avoid using these natural remedies when you are pregnant, breastfeeding, taking anti-coagulant drugs, or suffering from a complicated condition. It is better to check with your doctors first.

Other than that, it is also important that you remember that in taking these remedies, although they are effective in themselves, you also have to maintain a balanced and healthy living. Actually, most of the ailments listed in this book are a result of a sedentary lifestyle and excessive/insufficient nutrients. Water is very important, too. In fact, water is an effective remedy, too. It can even be considered the most natural of all remedies.

With these things in mind, I hope that you will be able to use all of the knowledge that you gained from this book and spread the wonder of nature's healing power to all.

Thank you and be well!

# Other Books By Dr Brad Turner

## Healing Honey For Beginners

Healing Honey For Beginners contains a complete and even very subtle information about honey- it's medical, aesthetic and its beautifying benefits. The entire book deals with the different uses of honey. This book is a complete guide for the people about honey and its several uses so that they can make the right decisions depending on their needs and stay thoroughly informed about the various benefits of honey.

We have often used honey for several purposes but most of us are completely unaware of the plethora of benefits honey has to offer to us. This book enlightens us with the most authentic and subtle information about honey and what it can be used for.

## Natural Antibiotics And Antivirals For Beginners

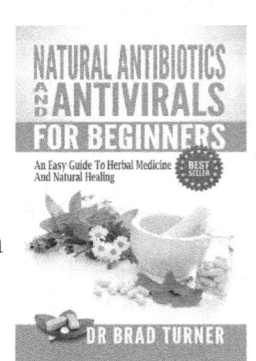

Herbs are among the first providers of medicines that had been used by our ancestors thousands of years ago. Since then, the world has developed sufficiently and new medicines made of various chemicals have been introduced to the people. This book specially focuses on the herbal medicinal antibiotics and antiviral. All the information given in the book has been very minutely researched and verified by professionals. So if you intend to start living by the cures of our ancestors, we suggest you order this book as soon as possible.

# Aromatherapy The Beginner's Guide

Frankincense. Peppermint. Eucalyptus. Lemon-grass. Lavender. Who knew that these are five of the must have essential oils? Dr. Brad Turner does—and we are blessed that he's chosen to share his knowledge and expertise in his latest book, ESSENTIAL OILS. So much has been written about using oils: as cures for everything from toothaches to acne; aromatherapy and even taken internally for whatever reason is popular that day.. To our own peril, we've discovered much of this information is false. Dr. Turner gains our trust immediately with his treatise: never ingest these essential oils. And that's the beginning of an author/reader relationship that will stand the test of time…and information, because Dr. Turner tells the truth. And that's the way we like it!

# Quit Smoking Naturally

On every literary corner, there's an expert on how to quit smoking. But very few of their theories stick. Every day the weary smoker is inspired to quit, only to have his/her hopes dashed yet again. *Quit Smoking Naturally* is the book that may set everyone free! The genius of this book is the straightforward approach and authentic voice that provides the facts, dispels the fallacies and motivates the smoker to do what they've never done before—succeed at quitting!

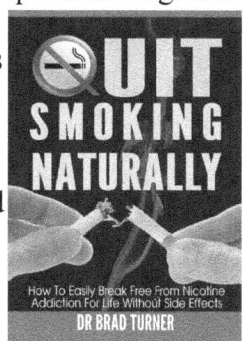

www.ingramcontent.com/pod-product-compliance
Lightning Source LLC
Chambersburg PA
CBHW070245290526
45789CB00004B/1768